Mental Health Week

Vincent A. Lanci

Disclaimer

I, Vincent A. Lanci, am not a medical professional and all content found in this book, *Mental Health Week*, is for informational purposes only.

The content in this book, *Mental Health Week*, is not intended to be a substitute for professional medical advice, treatment, or diagnosis.

Always seek the advice of qualified individuals, including your physician or contacting healthcare providers, with any inquiries related to a medical condition.

Never delay or disregard seeking professional medical advice because of something you have read in this book, *Mental Health Week*.

Meet the Author

Vincent A. Lanci is doing his part to remove the stigma associated with mental health. Following up his third book, *Mr. Lanci Talks Mental Health,* he is continuing to help others improve their mental well-being. *Mental Health Week* is the go-to book for students to level up their mental health.

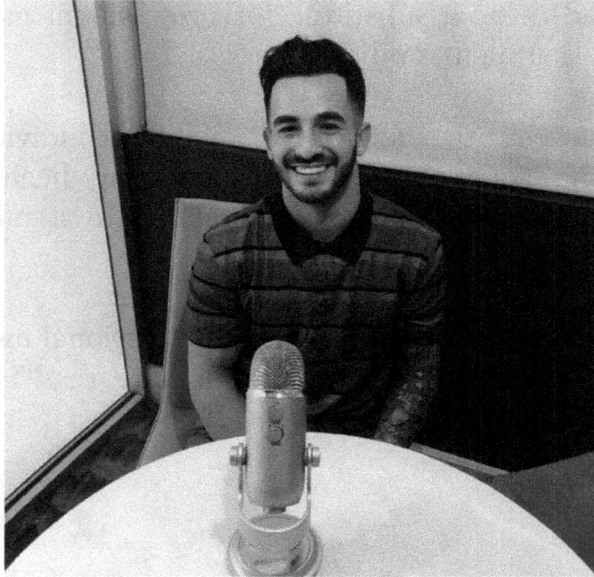

Acknowledgements

For my fourth book, I am going to acknowledge you. Thank you for making your mental health a priority.

Table of Contents

Preface

Hello class! My name is Mr. Lanci, teacher at *Never Give Up School*. We are a week away from summer break. Before I can send my class to middle school, I have an exciting week planned for their last week of school.

All of the students at our school have heard of *Mental Health Week*, but only the students in my class get to attend. Buckle up for an unforgettable and magical ride.

By joining us on our adventure, you are going to learn how to live a happy and healthy life, all about mental health, ways to take care of it, and improve it... all during *Mental Health Week*!

This resource contains information you may not know that will help you feel your best.

When I was 21 years old, I suffered a Traumatic Brain Injury (TBI). At first, there was speculation from the doctors as to whether I would make it through the initial night. As I remained alive, their concerns switched to whether I would ever be able to go to the bathroom on my own, walk, or talk properly again.

Over time, I began recovering from this horrific event, and quickly learned that I needed to make my mental health a priority. I want to help you do the same by sharing this book.

Join me and some of my favorite mental health experts in learning some tips that are sure to make a difference in your life!

To visit Vincent A. Lanci's website, visit: https://www.VincentALanci.com/

To purchase Vincent A. Lanci's first book, Left for Dead: A Story of Redemption, visit: https://www.VincentALanci.com/

To purchase Vincent A. Lanci's second book, How to Transform Your Mindset When the Norm is Changed, visit: https://www.VincentALanci.com/

To purchase Vincent A. Lanci's third book, Mr. Lanci Talks Mental Health, visit: https://www.VincentALanci.com/

To listen to Vincent A. Lanci's Podcast, *A Mental Health Break*, visit: https://amentalhealthbreak.buzzsprout.com/

To listen to Vincent A. Lanci's Podcast, *That Entrepreneur Show*, visit: https://www.dictionary.com/browse/entrepreneur

Monday Morning

It is that time of year. On the cusp of summer break, all of the students have grand plans for their time away from the classroom.

Last summer break was abnormal, and the students did not have much to celebrate. The 2020 Global Covid Pandemic swept across the world, but as restrictions have been lifted, the students are anxious to make up for lost time.

Before *Never Give Up School* releases its students for the summer, there is an event that Mr. Lanci's students have the opportunity to attend.

"I can't wait for summer break but am so excited for *Mental Health Week*," James texts to Grayson. "What do you think Mr. Lanci has planned for us?"

"Mr. Lanci has been talking about this week all year long! I am not sure what he has in store for us, but I know we are going to have a lot of fun and learn a lot about mental health," Grayson responds as he is putting on his pajamas.

"I have a friend who was in Mr. Lanci's 5th grade class last year and he said something happens with magic! He said whatever happened is a secret he can't share, but that I will understand what he means after the week is over. See you tomorrow, James."

The 2021-2022 school calendar is on its last page.

What a memorable year it has been. The students have learned a lot, had a lot of fun, and made lifelong friends over the course of the year. The students are experiencing many emotions.

While the students are excited that it is the final week of school, Mr. Lanci, however, is the opposite. He loves coming to school each day and helping his students prepare for their futures.

Each year, Mr. Lanci finishes his curriculum a week early to reward his students with an unforgettable last week before summer. *Mental Health Week* involves learning two things: all things mental health and the school's *biggest* secret. The *Magic Track* is a myth to most, but not to those who have had Mr. Lanci as a teacher.

Mr. Lanci has spent all weekend preparing for the last week of school with the help of School Security Guard, Stump. He aims to leave his students with one memory they will never forget, not only because it was fun, but because they were introduced to the world of mental health.

The importance of mental health has always been overlooked and has stigma attached to it. Now more than ever, Mr. Lanci wants to help his students thrive again after the 2020 Global Covid Pandemic. After this week, the students will be equipped with the tools

4

and strategies needed to live a healthy and fulfilling life.

He could not sleep all night due to pure excitement and arrived at school two hours early on the final Monday of the school year. Even after preparing for *Mental Health Week* all weekend, he still had four boxes to unpack from his car. He grabbed two and began walking to his classroom.

Stump, sitting at the entrance of the parking lot, greets Mr. Lanci at the door. "Do you think your students are ready for *Mental Health Week?*"

Stump, holding the door for Mr. Lanci, smiles as Mr. Lanci says, "The students are definitely looking forward to it. It is going to be a magical week. 2020 was a year that affected all of our mental health and this week will help them feel their best again. Thank you for helping me set up."

As Mr. Lanci puts his key into the classroom door, he hears someone's voice in the distance.

Connor, walking as fast as he can down the hallway, emphatically yells, "It is *Mental Health Week!*"

As the two enter the classroom, Mr. Lanci stops to glance around the room. He is incredibly proud of all that his students have accomplished over the year. For a moment, Connor notices him just smiling as he looks at their end-of-year projects.

Moments after entering the classroom, a second student has arrived early, too.

"Paul, it is great to see you looking forward to *Mental Health Week*. Would you like to help Connor and I bring in the final two boxes from the car?"

Mr. Lanci and his two students make a right out of the classroom and walk through the double doors to the parking lot. Stump gives high fives to both students as they walk past.

In a cheerful mood, Mr. Lanci glances over at his students and says, "Paul, did you know we are improving our mental health right now?"

"How are we improving our mental health? We are just walking," replies Paul.

"Exactly, Paul. We will talk more about this during the week, but nature, exercise, and socializing can all improve our mental health." As Mr. Lanci finishes previewing components of our mental health, he unlocks his car.

Connor notices the boxes are labeled, "Thursday" and "Friday". He curiously asks, "What's in these boxes, Mr. Lanci?"

Mr. Lanci smiles and says, "I can't tell you until Thursday and Friday, Connor. This is going to be an unforgettable week."

Connor and Paul each grab a box while Mr. Lanci helps Ms. Amorillo carry the objects she is holding. She is the teacher in the classroom next door and arrived at school at the same time.

Stump, holding the door open, smiles in joy as he is excited for the students to experience *Mental Health Week*.

Entering the classroom, the students place the two boxes next to Mr. Lanci's desk.

"Connor, how did getting some fresh air and taking a walk make you feel?" asks Mr. Lanci.

"I feel relaxed and ready to tackle the day, Mr. Lanci," Connor enthusiastically replies.

As the two students sit down at their desks, the rest of the students start entering the classroom.

Mr. Lanci feels like a child on the morning of a holiday. He is eager for his entire class to arrive so he can introduce the first day of this weeklong adventure.

At the end of each school year, Mr. Lanci takes his students on a five-day adventure to teach them about why mental health is important. When he was in college, he suffered a brain injury called a "Traumatic Brain Injury," or "TBI." A TBI is when damage to your brain changes the way it works. This injury affects everyone differently with symptoms that can range from mild to severe.

Ever since he began recovering from this injury and started teaching, he makes sure to teach his students about their brain's health, or mental health.

As Mr. Lanci prepares to take attendance, he notices the children expressing themselves uniquely and in a fun way.

He encouraged his students to wear clothes that make them happy for their last week together. One of the many ways to improve our mental health is to do things that make us happy, so it only felt right.

Austin and Bryson wore their Yankees hats to school, while Molly and Charlotte have their bathing suits on as they are headed to the beach after school.

Mr. Lanci continues to smile and glances around the room. He believes that it is time to take attendance. This is the largest class Mr. Lanci has ever had. *Never Give Up School* lost a lot of teachers for different reasons related to the 2020 Global Covid Pandemic.

Some of the remaining teachers were upset about a larger class size, but not Mr. Lanci. He relished the opportunity to teach additional students because even more children would be introduced to the world of mental health.

Ever since he began teaching at *Never Give Up School*, his average class size had been 23 students each year. Post-pandemic, he proudly has 37 students enrolled in his class for the 2021-2022 school year.

As Mr. Lanci finishes cleaning off his glasses, he looks at the class and begins, "Please stand up and do one jumping jack after I call out your name.

Brianna, Connor, Lily Mae, Lily Rose, James, Grayson, Jada Joy, Sophia, Olivia, Jackson, Shane, Riley, Elly, Cameron, Bryson, Moses, Paige...

... (silence) Paige? Is Paige here?

"I spoke to Paige last night. She went to the Raiders game with her mom yesterday and will not be back until tonight," says Gab.

Nicole added, "I wish Paige were here today!"

"We all do," Mr. Lanci continues. "Make sure to tell her all about how today goes. Please do your jumping jacks, Gab and Nicole.

Austin, Molly, Paul, Charlotte, Anthony, Jeff, Jill, Pete, Samantha, Zach, Mark, Dana, Christina, Michael, Dakota, Luke, Amanda, and Matthew."

Mr. Lanci leaves his desk and walks to the front of the classroom to introduce today's lesson.

"Today is the day! It is finally the Monday of *Mental Health Week* and I have been looking forward to this day for two years. Last year was the first year since I started teaching that my students did not get to experience this adventure because of the 2020 Global Covid Pandemic. It is great to see everyone physically healthy.

Before we begin our final week, I have a few questions for all of you. When was the last time you went to the doctor to get a checkup?"

Lily Mae, who always actively participates in class, is the first to answer, "I went the day before Halloween."

"I went the day before school started," Anthony added.

Mr. Lanci addresses the class while pointing to his teeth. "When was the last time you went to the dentist?" He points to Shane and Jill, both raising their hands.

Jill quickly answers first, "I went during the holiday break last year with my brother." Shane followed her answer with, "Right near my birthday."

Mr. Lanci loves how his students are taking turns contributing even though it is still early in the day. Most days, his students are still tired until an hour or two passes. Not for *Mental Health Week,* though!

He adds, "We all have a physical health. We go to the doctor for checkups and when we are sick. We all have a dental health. We go to the dentist for checkups and for teeth problems. We also have a mental health."

Mr. Lanci notices Riley ready to participate with her hand up. "What is mental health?"

"This is how healthy our brain and mind are. Our mental health affects how we feel, think, and act each day," says Mr. Lanci.

He continues, "When something does not feel normal, we always get checked, right?"

His students simultaneously nod their heads up and down.

Mr. Lanci leaves the front of the room and begins walking around the classroom. "The same needs to go for our mental health. Maybe thinking about it like this will help. When we break a bone in our bodies, we take time to heal.

We also need to take time to heal when we feel something is not normal with our mental health. If we experience mental health problems, our behavior, mood, and thinking can change.

If you feel there may be a problem with your mental health, do not worry. Mental health challenges are common and there are a lot of ways to fully recover. Never be afraid to speak to an adult you trust about how you are feeling because they can help you get the help you need.

You will learn how to live a happy and healthy life, all about mental health, ways to take care of it, and improve it, all during *Mental Health Week*! Please stand up and form a single-file line in alphabetical order. We are heading to the *Magic Track*.

Spot Check #1: What should you do if you are not feeling mentally healthy?

Sophia whispers to Olivia in line, "I thought the *Magic Track* was fake!"
Olivia tilts her head towards Sophia and whispers back, "I had a feeling it was real."

The whole school has heard of *Mental Health Week*. As Mr. Lanci's class walks through the halls, students in other classrooms smile and wave, wishing they could join in on the activities.

The students follow Mr. Lanci down the hallway towards the cafeteria. He suddenly stops at the cafeteria doors. He cracks the doors openly slowly to make sure no one is still eating morning breakfast.

Mr. Lanci smiles at the students and says, "The coast is clear!"

He holds the door open for his students to enter the cafeteria and says, "Please stay in a single-file line and stand next to the lunch table in front of the wall with the school flag hanging down."

Mr. Lanci follows the final student into the cafeteria to the lunch table with his classmates. Stump, following Mr. Lanci's class, locks the cafeteria doors behind them.

Mr. Lanci has given out five clues throughout the school year on what to expect during *Mental Health Week*. By the end of the week, his students will finally understand what each of the five clues mean.

"Can James, Connor, Grayson, Brianna, and Jada Joy please step forward. Did each of you bring your clue to school today?" Mr. Lanci asked.

All at once, the students shake their heads up and down.

Please read your clues to the class. The students decide to read the clues in alphabetical order. Brianna looks around at her classmates and delivers the first clue.

"There is a health besides physical health."

"Six guests will visit us during our last week of school."

"Magic is real."

"There is more than one track at our school."

"We will leave school, without leaving school, five times, during our last week of school."

After Jada Joy delivers the final clue, Mr. Lanci walks to the front of the lunch table and asks for three volunteers to come to the front.

Jackson, Cameron, and Elly quickly volunteered. "Class, please walk ten steps to the left of the lunch table. Jackson, Cameron, Elly, and I need to move this table to the right of the school flag on the wall."

Mark and Christina look at each other in confusion.

Once the table is moved, Jackson jokingly whispers to Cameron, "That was easy!"

Mr. Lanci takes down the school flag and folds in neatly on a neighboring table.

The students all point at the wall. There is a hidden door labeled, "Storage Closet," behind where the flag was. Mr. Lanci props the door to stay open.

As Mr. Lanci looks around at his students, he notices all of them have their jaws dropped! They are all surprised while also feeling puzzled and excited.

"I know this is a lot to take in. Enjoy the moment. The *Magic Track* is a secret you are now trusted to keep. There are five stations at the track. You will find out what makes the track magical at each station you go to," Mr. Lanci thrillingly adds.

"In alphabetical order, form a line at the Storage Closet. When it is your turn to stand in front of the Storage Closet, clap three times, and the door will open for one person at a time. Remember to hurry. The door only stays open for five seconds at a time.

When you walk through, please stand in a circle by the water fountain that is in the shape of a brain. This is *Mental Health Week*, after all," instructs Mr. Lanci.

Learning Checkpoint #1: Describe what mental health means to you.

Learning Checkpoint #2: Describe the shirt you would wear during Mental Health week and why you chose to wear it.

Monday Afternoon

The Magic Track was created by Mr. Lanci, six of his friends, or *Mental Health Week's* experts, and Principal Vaughn, after he suffered a Traumatic Brain Injury. To the surprise of the students, these experts are waiting to greet the class at the *Magic Track*.

These experts travel to Tampa, Florida for each *Mental Health Week*. They travel from all around the country to do their part in teaching children vital mental health topics and tools.

Although the experts only join the class on their day of *Mental Health Week,* they always come in for introductions on Monday, too.

These seven adults are smiling just as big as the students.

Mr. Lanci looks at the experts and says, "Thank you all for traveling here. It is great to see each one of you. Together, we are going to deliver a *Mental Health Week* like never before!

Please introduce yourselves to our students with your name, where you traveled from, and which day you will be leading the class."

"Mr. Jon Infeld, Edgewater, New Jersey. I will be your first expert."

"Dr. Richard Boccio, Miami, Florida. I will be back later this afternoon."

"Ms. Chris Helene Bridge, Houston, Texas. I will see you on Tuesday."

"Dr. Carlos Garcia, Tampa, Florida". I will see all of you on Wednesday."

"Mr. James Durand, East Northport, New York". I will be back on Thursday morning."

"Mr. Tony Alexander, Houston, Texas". I am looking forward to rejoining the class when I come back Thursday afternoon."

Mr. Lanci follows up with, "I will be your expert on our final day together this Friday. Before *Mental Health Week* is officially underway, our experts each baked their own dish for us to have a family style lunch together. We are going to save all of our questions until we see them again. Let's eat.

The class yells together, "Thank you experts!"

Each year, it is important to Mr. Lanci to make sure the students have a big meal before they start the final week of school. They are going to need the energy.

Paul is a food enthusiast and loves to watch cooking shows at home. He looks at Mr. Lanci, with a half-smile and asks, "I can ask questions about food though, right?"

"Of course, Paul. They are happy to help."

The students were starving and did not want to wait any longer to begin *Mental Health Week*. They ate their food in record time!

As everyone finishes eating, Mr. Lanci looks at the experts and says, "Thank you all for stopping by to say hello and meet my students. I look forward to seeing you on your day."

The students are looking out at an indoor track with five stations. Each station is set up differently and all have drawn the interest of the students.

Zach also notices the numbers "1", "2", "3", "4", and "5" are in big circles around the track. He whispers what he sees to Michael and both students are eager to begin.

Dana raises her hand and says, "Mr. Lanci, why are we at a track for mental health week?"

"Great question, Dana. Connor, Paul. Would one of you mind sharing what you learned about walking before school started?" follows Mr. Lanci.

Connor quickly shares, "Paul and I took a walk this morning and lifted some boxes. I feel better mentally and am thinking more clearly."

"Thank you for sharing, Connor. Mr. Jon Infeld is going to start *Mental Health Week*. As a Health teacher, he is going to further explain why we are walking the track to improve our mental health, along with the benefits exercise and a healthy diet have on our mental health.

Mr. Infeld walks towards the class and says, "Happy Monday! I am honored to start your final week of school. I have a great time here each year. Mr. Lanci was one of my roommates at The University of Tampa and I moved back to New Jersey after graduating.

We are going to walk the first 1/5 of the track to my station and sit down on the track when I stop walking.

The enthusiasm is evident as the class merrily follows Mr. Infeld.

"Let's stop here. We walk the track during *Mental Health Week* because of its benefits. Walking is important for our mental health because it makes us feel good and keeps us healthy.

Additional benefits of walking include making us feel happier, less stressed, more alert, and ready to make decisions.

Whenever we go walking, we get to see new things. Nature, cars, maybe meet a new friend walking along the way. Walking can be social, too. We can go walking with our friends, family, and pets.

Being social has many benefits for our mental health and Mr. Durand will discuss that in more detail when he comes back on Thursday.

Walking is a type of exercise. As you have learned so far, exercise is not only important for our physical health, but our mental health, too."

Gab is curious how exercising can improve her mental health, so she asks, "Are there any other reasons why exercise is important for our mental health?"

Mr. Infeld replies, "When we exercise, a lot of good things happen.

Exercising helps us develop healthy habits, sleep better, and keeps us healthy.

Class, please choose a partner. It is time to have fun and exercise. We will play a game called, "I Go, You Go."

With a smile on Lily Rose's face, she enthusiastically says, "I love that game!"

Mr. Infeld is thrilled to play this game with Mr. Lanci's class because his students in New Jersey love this game. He begins by showing the students correct form for pushups and sit-ups.

He starts by giving the direction, "Whichever exercise I do, copy me. I would like you to repeat after me.

Ready, set, go!

Let's start with ten pushups."
Walking around the room, Mr. Lanci notices Jeff using perfect form and shouts, "You are doing an awesome job, Jeff."

As Mr. Infeld and the class finish their pushups, he continues his instructions with, "Excellent job, class. Next let's do ten sit-ups."

Mr. Lanci continues to walk around the station and monitor the students. He notices all of the students are almost finished doing their pushups and sit-ups.

As the students complete their final exercise, Mr. Infeld also notices the children becoming fatigued.

"Amazing job, kids. Mr. Lanci, your class is awesome," says Mr. Infeld. He adds, "Let's break for a few minutes, grab a cup of water, and bowl of fruit on the table straight ahead."

Luke has always been a healthy eater. He asks, "Why is eating healthy important for our mental health?"

Mr. Infeld explains, "When we eat healthy, we are making our bodies and brains healthier.

Healthy food gives us the vitamins and minerals we need to stay healthy.

If we eat too much unhealthy food, we can become overweight, sick, or depressed. Dr. Boccio will teach you more about depression this afternoon.

A healthy diet means eating healthy foods. Who would like to tell me what their favorite fruit or vegetable is?"

"I have a banana every morning," says Samantha. Dakota adds, "I love apples."

Dakota is enjoying this lesson very much. He continues to participate, asking, "Mr. Infeld, why are you so passionate about health and exercise?"

Mr. Infeld takes a deep breath and shares, "Mr. Lanci and I both suffered a Traumatic Brain Injury. We did not get injured at the same time, but we helped each other get through them. We had to work hard to recover from our injuries and now both work to raise awareness to help others improve their mental health.

You have all been doing great so far. Now, raise your hands if you are ready for the first magical part of our adventure!"

All the students immediately raise their hands while Matthew is also jumping up and down.

When it comes time for magic each day, the class will need to leave the station area they are at and walk back to the track.

Zach made an astute observation earlier. He noticed five numbers in circles spread out across the track. Those are magic circles and where the magic happens! "Our track is unique and split into five sections," explains Mr. Lanci. "For the *Magic Track* to work, all of the students must stand in the middle of the circle. We are closest to "#1" on the track today because it is the first day of *Mental Health Week*.

When you come back tomorrow, you will be at Tuesday's station and closest to #2 on the track."

"The numbers are for which day of the school week it is!" Moses shouts.

"You are a very smart boy, Moses. Great observation," Mr. Lanci commends Moses.

He continues, "Once we are all standing in the middle of the circle and clap our hands three times, we will magically appear at a new location.

Amanda and Dana simultaneously shout, "Mr. Lanci. Where are we going first?"

"You will find out in three claps from now. Dr. Boccio will be waiting for us there to start our final activity. Say thank you to Mr. Infeld," Mr. Lanci follows.

The class runs to their first expert and gives him a giant hug.

As the students walk to the center of the circle, Mr. Lanci instructs the class. "Let's clap all together now.

Ready. Set. Let's clap."

1 clap.
2 claps.
3 claps.

POOF.

"Welcome everyone!" Dr. Boccio cheerfully says. He is wearing his scrubs and has a lot of new information to share with the students.

"I am an Emergency Resident Doctor not too far from here. My flight from Miami was less than one hour long. My job is to help people feel better. Mr. Lanci and I graduated both high school and college together. Some of you will be lifelong friends, too.

How did you enjoy your first experience with magic?

Brianna screams, "That was the coolest thing I have ever done!"

"I am happy to hear that. Mr. Lanci wanted to save the last hour of class for my session. Welcome to Bayshore Boulevard," Dr. Boccio says. "Please pass around this sunblock before we start our session."

The class has magically appeared at *Magic Location #1*. This secret location is on Bayshore Boulevard in Tampa. To be precise, the students have appeared outside of the grocery store on the Boulevard.

Bayshore Boulevard is the longest continuous sidewalk in the world. It overlooks the bay and is a sight for sore eyes. Dr. Boccio and the class will walk 20-minutes to the water table he set up before the students arrived. Afterwards, they will begin their walk back to *Magic Location #1*.

"As we walk along the sidewalk, we are going to first discuss why it is important to stay hydrated.

All living things need to drink water to survive. The body and brain need water to function. Water makes up half of our body weight and gives us energy."

Dr. Boccio continues, "We cannot live without water for more than a few days.

When we do not have enough water, our brains do not work correctly and slow down.

If we become dehydrated, we can experience mental health challenges, like depression and anxiety."[1]

Luke, normally quiet in class, raises his hand and asks, "Dr. Boccio, what is anxiety?"

"Great question," responds Dr. Boccio. "Anxiety is having worry and fear. It can also change our eating and sleeping patterns, moods, or behaviors."

Paige raises her hand next and asks, "...and what was that word you said that started with the letter D? I heard Mr. Infeld use it earlier."

"Ah, another great question," Dr. Boccio talking while walking. "Remember class, it is normal to feel sad once and a while because sometimes unhappy things happen in life. Depression is when we are sad or in a bad mood for a really long time.

Remember, always tell a parent, guardian, or teacher when you are not feeling normal. If something has changed with your sleep, energy, or diet, talk to an adult you are comfortable with. They want to help.

Ah, I sure am thirsty," Dr. Boccio says. "Let's stop at the water table coming up on the right of us and take five minutes to cool off under the trees. I will set a timer on my phone."

As the class is enjoying the shade and cold water, Mr. Lanci addresses the class, "I would like to share more benefits to walking outside.

An easy way to improve our mood is by getting natural sunlight. It sounds simple, but it is incredibly effective.

After applying sunscreen, do your best to get outside and enjoy fifteen minutes of sunshine each day. The natural sunlight synthesizes Vitamin D, which can improve our moods. This is one reason why we are walking outside this afternoon.

Dr. Boccio's timer sounds, and the class starts walking back towards *Magic Location #1*.

Dr. Boccio restarts the conversation, "While enjoying natural sunlight, it is a great time to focus on each of our senses. When we use our five senses, it allows us to focus on what is around us.

As depression narrows our focus, expanding our view using our senses helps us appreciate the world we live in. When times get tough, step outside to focus on your surroundings. This simple exercise will help us relax.

Who knows what our senses are? Anyone can answer."

Mr. Lanci and Dr. Boccio hear,

"Smell and touch."
"Taste!"
"Sound and sight."

Dr. Boccio claps and says, "Well done, Moses, Amanda, and Cameron. If we use our senses, we can better focus on what is around us. Using our senses allows us to relax and appreciate our surroundings.

Let's take one minute to focus on our senses. I will set another timer."

Mr. Lanci is extremely proud of his class for actively engaging with both guests so far. They are paying immense attention and asking relevant questions.

"Does everyone feel relaxed right now?" asks Dr. Boccio.

The class happily says together, "We feel amazing mentally and physically!"

The class is approaching *Magic Location #1* yet are full of energy like the day has not begun yet. "The last topic I would like to introduce is one more challenge students may experience mentally," begins Dr. Boccio.

It is a long name, but there is an abbreviation, don't worry. This mental health challenge is called, "Attention Deficit Hyperactive Disorder," or ADHD.

Students struggling with ADHD may have trouble focusing, sitting still, or act impulsively. What I am about to say to you next you have already heard today and will hear again this week. I cannot stress it enough.

If you ever feel like something is not normal, there is no need to panic. Talk to a trusted adult and everything will be okay. Tough times do not last, but you will!

This session went so fast. It was great to meet all of you."

Dr. Boccio waves goodbye as the students are arriving at *Magic Location #1*.

Altogether, the students begin clapping.

1 clap.
2 claps.
3 claps.

POOF.

Learning Checkpoint #3: What are two mental health benefits from walking?

Learning Checkpoint #4: Describe "Anxiety" in your own words.

Tuesday Morning

There was a lot going through the minds of Mr. Lanci's students when they left school yesterday.

They learned many things on Day 1 of *Mental Health Week*. Maintaining a healthy diet, staying hydrated, exercising, using our senses, and getting natural sunlight are all ways to stay mentally healthy. They also learned about the biggest secret their school has to offer.

Although it would be a challenging task for his students, Mr. Lanci was confident they would be able to keep the *Magic Track* a secret. He has never had a class that could not keep this mystical secret.

Each expert Mr. Lanci brings in has a special relationship with him. Dr. Boccio has been his friend for fifteen years. Today's guest is the illustrator in Mr. Lanci's third book, *Mr. Lanci Talks Mental Health*. The students are going to love her. She is one of the most creative, caring, and inspiring people Mr. Lanci knows.

Ms. Chris Helene Bridge is an award-winning author, artist, and literacy advocate. Her creative work continues to make a difference to people worldwide. For Tuesday's lesson, she will lead one session in the morning and another in the afternoon.

Ms. Bridge has *Magic Station #2* set up like an art studio. There are 37 easels and stools to sit on. Each student's palette has so much paint on it that they could paint forever!

Paige has returned to school after being out yesterday. Nicole and Gab have been telling her about all of the fun they had and information they learned.

The students are wearing their favorite shirts again today. They are really enjoying showing their shirts off to their friends. Sophia is wearing a milk-colored shirt because that is her favorite color, while Olivia has her favorite TV show character on her shirt. Of course, Paige is wearing her new Raiders jersey.

Ms. Bridge is walking around the station as she is almost ready to begin. She overhears Lily Mae and James talking more about Mr. Infeld and Dr. Boccio's sessions.

Yet to reintroduce herself from Monday morning, Ms. Bridge asks Lily Mae, "What is one thing you took away from yesterday's sessions?"

"I asked my daddy to buy me a big water bottle so I can stay hydrated. See, it's pink and blue," she responds and holds the water bottle up.

"Thank you for sharing. Good morning Kids," Ms. Bridge greets the class.

"Once again, I am Ms. Bridge and thank you for having me. I have written many books for children your age."

Elly rapidly raises her hand after Ms. Bridge speaks. "We read your book, *Read to Me*, in September. Mr. Lanci said we would meet you, but we didn't know it would be at the *Magic Track*!"

Ms. Bridge can do nothing but smile. "I created that book to inspire the love of reading in students just like you.

For the morning session, we are going to talk about how mental health and creativity are related.

Everybody is a creative being.
We are all creators.
We are all creative people.
What makes us unique is that we all use different methods to create with.
Every part of our brain is programmed to create in a different way.

A writer creates with their words.
A chef creates with their food.

What are some ways you like to act creatively?"

Bryson and Jada Joy are quick to raise their hands.

"I like to play with clay," says Bryson.

"I really love to draw," adds Jada Joy.

Ms. Bridge follows up with, "Those are two excellent ways to express ourselves creatively. Now let's talk about what mental health and creativity have in common.

Mr. Lanci told me Dr. Boccio introduced anxiety and depression yesterday. When we act in creative ways, we lower both of those things. Creativity puts us in a happy mood.

I want to teach all of you a cool fact. We have around 60,000 thoughts each day. If we are having thoughts we do not want to have, being creative can take our mind to a happy place. Creativity calms our minds."

"Did you say 60,000?" surprisingly asks Riley.

"I did!" as Ms. Bridge smiles back. "Some days are good days, and some days are bad days. It is okay to have a bad day. If you are having a bad day in the future, I challenge you to get creative.

We are now going to pick up the paintbrushes in front of our easels and act in a creative way before we break for lunch.

Using only three colors on your palettes, think creatively and draw something that puts a smile on your face. It can be anything.

You only have five minutes though! Mr. Lanci, please start the timer.

3.
2.
1.
Let's get creative."

Spot Check #2: List and describe two things you learned on Monday of *Mental Health Week*.

Mr. Lanci and Ms. Bridge walk around the station, both so proud of what they are seeing. To their surprise, all of the students used one common color: blue! Blue and gold are the school colors at *Never Give Up School*.

As the timer sounds, Ms. Bridge gains the students attention by clapping. "Well done, everyone. I need three volunteers to share their creation. Please raise your hand if you would like to share your painting.

Charlotte, Michael, and Austin quickly raise their hands.

Charlotte proudly holds up a picture of her with her dog.
Michael draws a picture of him and his father.

Austin shares his picture of him at a Yankees game.

Mr. Lanci gives Austin a high-five as Ms. Bridge says, "Class, please put your paintings near your backpacks and break for lunch. Mr. Lanci told me you were all bringing your own lunch today. You can eat anywhere you would like as long as it is in this station. See you in one hour."

Learning Checkpoint #5: Name one way in which you create and what the creation will be.

Learning Checkpoint #6: Name at least one mental health benefit from expressing yourself creatively.

Tuesday Afternoon

Christina finished lunch early to talk more with Ms. Bridge. Similarly, to Charlotte, she also painted her dog and wanted to show the expert.

The class has not even finished Day 2 of *Mental Health Week*, yet the students have already learned so much about mental health. Ms. Bridge began her session with creativity and has another fun-packed and informative lesson planned for this afternoon. There may even be some magic!

By introducing the mental health benefits creativity provides, Ms. Bridge has provided the students with another tool to improve their mental well-being.

As the rest of the class finishes eating, the students begin throwing out their garbage and cleaning up. Normally, the students choose to relax for a few minutes after lunch before normally heading out to the playground, but not during *Mental Health Week*. As soon as Ms. Bridge offers the idea of taking a walk before beginning her afternoon session, the students jump up from where they are eating.

"We are going to walk a lap around the track to digest and feel ready for our afternoon session," starts Ms. Bridge.

"Let's have some fun as we walk. Let's take turns saying what we brought in to eat today.

Olivia says, "Walking sounds like a great idea. Dr. Boccio and Mr. Infeld taught us how important it is."

"Well done, Olivia," Mr. Lanci replies.

The students joyfully begin walking around the track. Some students are focused on the curtains guarding the secrets behind Wednesday, Thursday, and Friday's stations, while the others are brainstorming new ways they can act creatively after school.

You can see the relationships among the students becoming stronger. There is a stronger sense of camaraderie, and the class is becoming a family!

"This week is special for many reasons. When I was a student at The University of Tampa, the classmates and adults that I was close with were my *Tampa Family*. I would love for you all to make lifelong friends, too, while learning all things mental health," Mr. Lanci continues.

Dakota shares what he ate for lunch first, shouting "I had a PB&J."
Lily Rose follows up by saying, "Me too. I love Peanut Butter and Jelly sandwiches."

As the students return to Ms. Bridge's station, they do not know what to expect for the afternoon session.

"Now that we are feeling reenergized, it is time for magic!" says Ms. Bridge.

Let's now walk to the track and get ready to clap."

1 clap.
2 claps.
3 claps.

POOF.

The class arrives at Ms. Bridge's choice for *Magic Location #2*. The students are now at her art studio in Texas! Her incredible work and books are spread out on the tables and easels throughout her studio. Her breathtaking paintings are also hanging on the walls.

Shane, one of Mr. Lanci's most creative students, is mesmerized as he looks around the studio.

Ms. Bridge begins, "When I first decided to become an artist, I needed to find a place to create. I fell in love with this studio right away."

Elly interrupts as she notices Ms. Bridge's book, *Read to Me*, "There is the book we read."

"Good eye, Elly! I am grateful students get to enjoy that book.

I am also grateful for all of the learning lessons I have had in this studio. Whether you are an artist, banker, or author, there is always a lot of learning involved. In anything we do, we need to work hard and practice. The next topic related to mental health that I would like to introduce is about being grateful.

Would anyone like to guess what being grateful means?" requests Ms. Bridge.

The class has a puzzled look on their faces, but Bryson tries anyway and says, "When we are really good at a task or activity. I'm great at sports."

"Thank you for participating, Bryson," replies Ms. Bridge. "You are correct! You are great at sports. This word has a different meaning, and I am glad I can teach all of you a new word."

Bryson always participates in Mr. Lanci's class. He has the confidence and ambition to accomplish large feats as he gets older.

After commending Bryson, Ms. Bridge continues, "I am going to share a few definitions of the word, grateful.

A warm or deep appreciation of kindness or benefits received.

An expression of gratitude.

Pleasing to the senses or mind.

After sharing these definitions, I would like to now ask for three volunteers to give an example of how they are grateful for something in their lives.

Please raise your hand if you would like to share an example," Ms. Bridge asks of the class.

Within seconds, the entire class has raised their hands. Ms. Bridge points at Pete, Riley, and Jackson.

Pete starts, "I am grateful for Samantha," as he blushes. Pete and Samantha have been boyfriend and girlfriend since their third year of school!

Riley answers second and says, "I am grateful for having a roof over my head."

Jackson follows with, "I am grateful for having food to eat each day."

Mr. Lanci and Ms. Bridge begin clapping their hands. "Well done class," Ms. Bridge says.

"There are many positive benefits to living a grateful life. They include less stress, depression, and anxiety, while also being happier. When we express genuine gratitude, our quality of sleep will also improve.

When we are grateful, we are creating a positive mindset. I challenge you to slow down and look around when thinking about things you are grateful for. The things we should be most grateful for are often right in front of us, not expensive items or objects.

I can think of two right now. One, it is a beautiful day. Second, we all are able to spend the day together. It was wonderful to meet you all.

I hope to see some of your creative works in the future. Have a great summer."

<u>Learning Checkpoint #7</u>: Describe what the being "grateful" means in your own words.

<u>Learning Checkpoint #8</u>: Name at least two benefits from expressing gratitude.

Wednesday Morning

The first two days of *Mental Health Week* have given the students a lot to think about. After this week ends, Mr. Lanci's goal is to have everyone consider their mental health as a top priority.

Mr. Lanci came in early to set up a healthy breakfast for his students to enjoy. To his surprise, the students have all arrived at school earlier than him today.

When school ended yesterday, Stump and Mr. Lanci's student, Paul, played a game of "Rock, Paper, Scissors". If Stump won, Paul would need to wear a Giants jersey to school, even though he is a Jets fan. If Paul won, Stump would need to come in one hour early each day to supervise the class until Mr. Lanci arrives. Paul is a classroom hero for winning this epic showdown.

Connor and Riley were anxious for school to start as they wanted to show their friends their clothes. Connor plays hockey so he decided to wear his team jersey. Riley is wearing a shirt she made in art class this year. She was inspired to wear it after spending the day with Ms. Bridge.

Brianna was doing the sit-ups she learned this week, and Samantha and Pete were talking about healthy foods they are going to try after *Mental Health Week* ends.

Stump holds the door open for Mr. Lanci and his class to make their way to the *Magic Track*.

Jeff, always intrigued, is curious about what today's adventure will be. Being curious, he glances around Wednesday's station. He notices an American flag, windows overlooking the Tampa Bay waters, and mats on the floor in the shape of a circle.

Seconds before Stump locks the doors to the cafeteria, Anthony arrives. Each day, Stump locks the cafeteria doors once the entire class leaves for their adventure to ensure the secret is kept safe.

As soon as Anthony arrives at the *Magic Track*, Mr. Lanci instructs the class to complete 10 sit-ups, eat breakfast, and to each sit on a mat.

As the school day is about to start, the students choose between yogurt and fruit to bring back to their mats.

For Wednesday's session, the class will meet an entrepreneur based right here in Tampa. Dr. Carlos Garcia is a Psychologist who owns his own practice. Who knows, maybe with a little magic, the students will get to see his office later.

"Earlier we spoke about how we go to the doctors and dentist office when we need to check our physical health," starts Mr. Lanci. "As we have learned this week, we also need to check on our mental health.

Please give a round of applause for my good friend, Dr. Carlos Garcia!"

The students stand up from sitting in a circle and, all together, clap as Dr. Garcia walks to the front of the station.

"Good morning and thank you for coming to my station. I am the owner and primary Psychologist at "Tampa Counseling and Wellness." My areas of expertise are areas you learned earlier this week. I help those who struggle with anxiety, depression, self-esteem, and motivation.

Each individual has a different and unique mental health. Students may choose to become my patient to maintain a positive mindset, while other kids may become my patient to gain a positive mindset.

I am also a veteran."

"What is a Veteran?" asks Molly.

Walking around the station, he replies, "Thank you for asking questions and engaging with me right away. A Veteran is someone who has served in a branch of military."

Mr. Lanci gives Dr. Garcia a handshake and looks at the class, "When you see a Veteran in uniform in public, make sure to thank them for their service. Veterans have fought to give us freedom."

Dr. Garcia begins, "I help children, just like all of you, every day as a Psychologist."

Mark asks, "What is a Psychologist?"

Dr. Garcia responds, with a smile on his face, "Wonderful question, Mark.

Psychologists are professionals in the mental health field. We specialize in studying the minds and behaviors of others. Two ways we help others is by improving their emotional skills and lowering the chance they experience symptoms of a mental health challenge.

As a Psychologist, I offer support, guidance, and compassion to others while helping them find their strengths.

Jeff, you noticed the beautiful view of the water. When I meet with students at my office, they find the view of Tampa Bay to be soothing. When we created the *Magic Track*, having a water view at my station was prioritized because of how much my own patients enjoy it.

Jada Joy follows up with, "Looking out at the water makes me feel calm."

"I feel the same way," Lily Mae replies.

Dr. Garcia continues to walk around the station. "I am glad you both said that. While we are relaxed, I would like to introduce breathwork to you.

Breathwork is when we can use breathing exercises to feel calmer and more relaxed. By practicing breathwork, we become more attuned with ourselves. Breathing is connected to our nervous system in our bodies. Our nervous system is in charge of the way we respond to things.

What are some situations that make you feel afraid, anxious, or uncomfortable?" Dr. Garcia asks the entire class.

"When I have a test at school," Cameron responds.

"When my mom shuts the lights off before bed," Grayson follows Cameron.

"I used to feel afraid when talking to Samantha!" Pete adds.

When we feel this way, breathing can shift the way our entire body functions. I know it can be scary and challenging to feel this way. Breathwork may also help you share how you are feeling more easily.

Spot Check #3: Describe what Dr. Garcia does at Tampa Counseling and Wellness in your own words.

Dr. Garcia continues, "As a class, we are going to do an exercise together and I encourage you to try this when times get tough. It will help you return to a "safe place.""

Mr. Lanci and Dr. Garcia hand out a piece of paper that explains the type of exercises the class is about to do. Dr. Garcia created this guide for students to have when they practice breathwork on their own.

"Gab, would you mind please teaching us the first exercise?" Mr. Lanci asks.

"Of course!" as Gab jumps up. She continues, "Belly Breathing. Belly breathing is when we deepen our breath. To do this, we simply expand our bellies while breathing in and flatten our bellies while we breathe out."

"Well done, Gab," said Dr. Garcia. He continues, "We are going to play a game together. Now, these mats are coming in handy, huh?

Mr. Lanci, would you mind giving instructions for our game while I pass out a book to each student?"

Amanda interrupts, "Oh man, are we reading today? I thought we were on a field trip?"

Mr. Lanci clears his throat and begins with, "Absolutely, Dr. Garcia. Amanda, we're not reading today, don't worry. You will find out what the books are for in just a second. Choose a partner and bring your mat next to theirs. Say "DONE!" when you are ready to move on."

The class eagerly screams, "DONE!", within seconds, and starts laughing. Mr. Lanci and Dr. Garcia smile, too.

Mr. Lanci begins, "The first step is to lay down on your mats next to each other.

Next, take the books Dr. Garcia passed out and place them on your stomachs.

Our goal in this game is to balance the book while we are breathing. Take a deep breath through your nose and see how large you can fill your stomach. Do not fill your stomach to the point where it hurts, though."

Dr. Garcia takes over giving instructions. "We are going to breathe out completely through our noses and that should push the air out of our stomachs. Watch the book go up and down with each breath. Have fun and grab your lunch from your backpacks after the game. We will break for lunch afterwards.

Learning Checkpoint #9: What is a therapist?

Learning Checkpoint #10: Describe at least two things you learned about breathwork in complete sentences.

Wednesday Afternoon

Dr. Garcia begins walking around his station as the students are wrapping up eating lunch. He has had just as much fun as the kids.

"It is time for a little magic to start the afternoon," says Dr. Garcia.
The students walk to the track and stand in the center of *Magic Circle #3*. With their faces glowing, they clap together three times.
1 clap.
2 claps.
3 claps.

POOF.

The class arrives at *Magic Location #3*. They have magically appeared at Dr. Garcia's office on Martin Luther King Blvd in Tampa.

"I have driven past your office a million times!" says Charlotte.
"So have I," follows Christina.

Dr. Garcia speaks next, "Who can remember the name of my company?"

Grayson almost immediately blurts out, "Tampa Counseling and Wellness." Grayson has an incredibly strong memory and is going to be very successful when he grows up.

As Riley walks throughout the office, she glances at the coffee table and sees Mr. Lanci's face. Dr. Garcia has Mr. Lanci's book, *Mr. Lanci Talks Mental Health*, on the table for patients to read while they are waiting. "Hey, I know that guy," Riley jokingly whispers to Connor.

Very pleased with how well the morning session went, Dr. Garcia is looking forward to talking about self-love and self-care. He holds a picture up to the class and says, "This is my best friend, Ellie, and me. She is supportive, dependable, and funny. Mr. Lanci's class has a superstar named Elly, too!

Lily Rose, if your best friend was here right now, what would you say to him or her?"

Lily Rose happily answers, "I will be there for them when they need me. I will also tell them that if they have a bad day, I will help cheer them up.

Dr. Garcia, impressed with her answer, follows with, "Great answer. Just as we are kind to the people in our lives, we need to treat ourselves the same way. It is important to love and care for ourselves, too.

It is important to fill our heads with thoughts that relax us, not make us worried or nervous. Words are very powerful and can lead us into either a healthy or unhealthy state.

Don't forget this: there is nothing wrong with having feelings. It is okay to feel sad, worried, or have butterflies in our stomachs. It is normal to have feelings and emotions.

Life can be like a rollercoaster sometimes. There are going to be highs and lows. It is okay to talk to someone if you need to.

It is okay to see someone if it will help.

I am here if you need me. Your parents were sent an email with each experts contact information, and I am only a phone call away.

Let's walk back to the front door of the office and clap our way home.

Thank you for a great session.

1 clap.
2 claps.
3 claps.

POOF.

Learning Checkpoint #11: Describe what self-love and self-care mean to you.

<u>Learning Checkpoint #12:</u> List and describe two emotions or feelings you enjoy and two emotions or feelings you dislike.

Thursday Morning

You guessed it. The whole class is not only filled with energy and enthusiasm but have all arrived before Mr. Lanci once again.

The students are having a pushup contest out in the field, anxiously awaiting Mr. Lanci's arrival.

Stump is keeping tally for each student, rooting them on like they were his own kids. Stump enjoys his time with the students as he does not have any kids of his own.

Anthony teases Stump, "I bet I can do more pushups than you!"

Stump jokingly replies, "You should have seen me when I was younger."

He waves at Mr. Lanci as he pulls in his parking spot. As he walks by with his briefcase, Stump whispers, "I gotta' tell you, Mr. Lanci. Even though I lost the Rock, Paper, Scissor's game, I feel like I won. I get to spend an extra hour with your awesome students each morning."

"Now you know how I feel every day. I love my job," responds Mr. Lanci.

Mr. Lanci is not alone this morning, however. He is with a man who the students have never seen before.

Nicole whispers to Sophia, "Do you think that is today's guest?"

"It has to be, Nicole!" Sophia excitingly says.

As Stump locks the doors to the cafeteria, Mr. Lanci has still not introduced the individual to the class. The students look like they are about to burst full of anticipation.

They have become infatuated with the topic of mental health. The entire class wants to keep learning and are participating more than ever before.

As the class is lining up at the Storage Closet, Zach looks at the experts and raises his hand. Mr. Lanci finally calls on Zach after making him wait a few seconds. "I think I have seen him in a picture in our classroom. Am I right? Is that today's expert?"

The experts do not say yes or no, but reply, "I am not sure!", instead. There is now even more anticipation among the students.

1 clap.
2 claps.
3 claps.

POOF.

As the class appears at the *Magic Track*, Jeff pulls the curtain to open Thursday's station. Mr. Lanci finally prepares to introduce today's guest. Zach was smart enough to have made an observation.

"Class, I would like to start by asking the class this question:

"On a scale of one to ten, how much do you appreciate and enjoy spending time with your school counselor?"

"11!", blurts out Mark.
"12!", says Molly.

Mr. Lanci high fives Mark and Molly and says, "I feel the same way. With that, I would like to introduce my counselor from when I was in elementary school, Mr. James Durand. We have stayed in touch over the years and I have also returned to my old school to speak at Leadership Day a few years ago.

Zach, great job recognizing him and, Mr. Durand, thank you for flying to Florida from New York for another *Mental Health* week."

Mr. Durand is ecstatic when greeting the class. "It is great to see you, Mr. Lanci. Class, thank you for spending the fourth day of *Mental Health Week* with me. I am happy to be in a place warmer than New York!"

Mr. Durand is going to teach the class about a few important topics they did not cover yet. There are many topics most do not think of right away when they are thinking about their mental health.

Mr. Durand takes a sip of his coffee and restarts, "Some of the things Dr. Garcia spoke about yesterday were loving and caring for ourselves. Similarly, we want to make sure we are a supportive and loving friend or family member so we can share our feelings when we need to. We want to surround ourselves with the same type of people."

Dana asks, "Why is sharing our feelings important for our mental health?"

"Interacting with others makes us happier and puts us in a better mood. It is an amazing way to feel better when things are not going well," follows Mr. Durand.

"It lowers the chance we feel depressed and alone. Talking with others is one way we support one another. When we are sad, it makes us feel less alone.

Raise your hand if you like to feel loved."

The whole class rapidly raises their hand.

Mr. Durand goes on to say, "Having a support group to count on is an important part of life. This can include supportive friends and family who we can talk to about the good and bad times in life.

Instead of keeping things to ourselves, it is important to talk to others about how we are feeling. Socializing also lowers the chance we feel depressed.

We have heard of independence and codependence. There is also something called interdependence. This is something that is right in the middle.

An example of interdependence can be a close personal relationship, like two best friends who are supportive of each other.

Mr. Lanci, who is supportive in your life?"

Mr. Lanci smiles and says, "My mother, father, and sister are very supportive of me. Even though I live over 1,000 miles away from them, when we see each other, it is as if nothing has changed. I can go to them for advice, and they help me feel better when I am overwhelmed.

Two of my most supportive friends are Alan and Daniel. We share ideas with each other and help one another see things from their point of view.

Mr. Durand stops Mr. Lanci and says, "I remember Daniel!"

"Yes, you do," replies Mr. Lanci.

"Class, I met Daniel in my Kindergarten class. You have already met another lifelong friend of mine, in

Dr. Boccio. Some of you will be friends forever. Isn't that awesome?

Dakota puts both thumbs up!

Mr. Lanci resumes, "Daniel is a lifelong friend and we have always supported each other.

Daniel and I often share ideas and talk in the outdoors. From sitting in one of our backyards, to taking walks in nature trails, it is always great to catch up with him."

Mr. Durand asks, "Did Alan go to elementary school with you, too?"

"Alan was one of my college roommates at The University of Tampa," says Mr. Lanci.

Similar to how Daniel and I share ideas in the outdoors, Alan and I sometimes sit on the couch for hours, just enjoying the conversation. By listening to someone else's point of view, we can understand things in a way we normally are not able to."

Mr. Durand follows up Mr. Lanci with, "Thank you for sharing, Mr. Lanci. I want to touch on one more topic before leaving today.

I would like to teach the class about self-awareness. It is a big word, but has a fun meaning. Self-awareness is what our minds think and bodies feel.

When we are hungry, our stomachs tell us we are hungry."

Jackson asks, "Is this like when I am feeling tired and my eyes get heavy, I know I am ready for bed?"

"Very good, Jackson. That is a great example," Mr. Durand adds.

Mr. Durand finishes with a big wave, "It looks like Mr. Lanci ordered pizza for us. Thank you, Mr. Lanci."

As the class is finishing their lunches, Mr. Lanci frantically says, "Oh! I almost forgot. Connor, Paul. Please come help me unpack the box labeled "Thursday" since you helped me carry it in on Monday. I brought both boxes to their respective stations before school today."

The boys walk towards Mr. Lanci and begin carefully removing the tape around the box.

It is photos, a yearbook, and class t-shirt from when he was in elementary school. He thought it would be fun to share these memories with his students on the day Mr. Durand visits. Certain memories last a lifetime.

"Feel free to come look at some of my memories from when I was your age. Take care, Mr. Durand."

The class waves goodbye and enjoys a second slice of pizza.

Learning Checkpoint #13: Describe either interdependence or codependence in your own words.

Learning Checkpoint #14: Describe at least one topic you can talk to your school counselor about if you need to.

Thursday Afternoon

The students are still nowhere near running out of energy.

Jackson and Cameron are wondering when something magical is going to happen.

Pete is over in the corner just stretching. He is more than ready to start walking again. He wants to participate in CrossFit exercises when he becomes big and strong.

Shane impatiently adds, "This week has been so much fun. We are ready when you are!"

The students were so busy wondering what Mr. Lanci has in store for them next that they did not hear their next guest walk in. A man tapped Mr. Lanci on the shoulder, catching him off-guard. Although off-guard, he is thrilled, and says, "Mr. Alexander, there you are. It is great to see you."

"I hit a lot a traffic on my way over from the amusement parks. I am a long way from Texas, so I want to make the most of my trip to Florida!" Mr. Alexander greets the class.

"I love going to the amusement parks," shouts James. "My family and I go a few times per year. Check out the shirt I am wearing. It is from my favorite ride."

"Thank you for sharing, James. Can I have one more volunteer tell me about their outfit today?" Mr. Alexander says to the class.

Elly raises her hand and looks at Mr. Alexander. "I am wearing a shirt with a penguin because it is my favorite animal."

"Elly, thank you for volunteering. I could not be more excited to meet another 5th grade class. My name is Mr. Tony Alexander and like Dr. Garcia, I am also an entrepreneur. I provide leadership to businesses around the country.

I am also both a Mental Health Advocate and Diversity, Equity, and Inclusion Advocate. Those are the causes I am passionate about. Can someone tell me something they are passionate about?

Michael quickly responds, "I am passionate about bringing food to homeless people."

"That is very admirable, Michael."

Since you have had to wait all day for some magic, I know how excited you must be. Let's get ready to go to *Magic Location #4*. Everyone, please follow me to the track. Please walk back to Wednesday's station and grab your yoga mats first.

As the students arrive to *Magic Circle #4* on the track, Sophia asks, "Are we doing the same thing as Wednesday?"

Mr. Alexander looks at Sophia and says, "New day, new information. You are going to learn about yoga and meditation, but we have to clap a few times first, right?!"

1 clap.
2 claps.
3 claps.

POOF.

Since the class had so much fun on their walk on Bayshore Boulevard, Mr. Lanci decided to plan another day where the students can go on a walk together. Only this time, they are at Henry B. Plant park next to The University of Tampa.

Spot Check #4: What was your biggest takeaway from Mr. Durand's time with you?

The exact place of *Magic Location #4* is at the fountain separating The University of Tampa and the park. Henry B. Plant Park overlooks Downtown Tampa and is on the Hillsborough River. It is filled with trees, smaller bodies of water, and a sidewalk throughout.

It is a beautiful day. The sun is shining and the birds are chirping. There are boats on the river and college students studying outdoors.

Mr. Lanci's class sets up their mats and the afternoon session begins as Christina asks, "So, what is a Mental Health Advocate?"

Mr. Alexander puts his thumbs up and says, "Great question. A Mental Health Advocate is someone who supports mental health.

I use my voice to raise awareness for the importance of mental health. I help other people become more mentally healthy and understand the basics about their mental health.

One way to improve our mental health is to meditate. Mr. Lanci said this park brought him a lot of peace and comfort when academics got difficult in college."

Mr. Lanci takes over, "Henry B. Plant Park is located directly next to the Macdonald-Kelce Library at The University of Tampa, so I was able to take walks as breaks from studying. I thought it would be the perfect place to take the class today.

Mr. Alexander continues, "Before we start, I want to teach you some things that meditating does. I wrote a few of those things on an index card so one of you students can read it to the class. Can a volunteer raise their hand please?"

Lily Mae is the first to do so and walks over to take the index card from Mr. Alexander.

Lily Mae reads, "Meditating does many positive things for our bodies, including improving our sleep, breathing, and ability to focus. It also helps us become less stressed and happier. This helps people struggling with anxiety."

Mr. Alexander follows Lily Mae's reading with, "Excellent job, Lily Mae."

Wiping the sweat off his forehead, he addresses the class. "Everyone look up at Lily Mae and I as we will begin together.

First, let's take five deep breaths. We want to be sitting still and as calm as possible when we meditate.

Make sure to focus on your breathing. In through the nose, out through the mouth. We will meditate for only two minutes as many of you are meditating for the first time. Try to relax.

Amanda and Michael look extremely relaxed and at ease as Mr. Lanci glances over the students.

As the alarm rings, Dakota calmly speaks to his classmates, "That was an amazing two minutes." "Excellent work everyone," Mr. Alexander follows.

"Time flies when you are having fun. We have 30 minutes left, and that is the perfect amount of time for our next activity. How many of you have heard of yoga?"

Half of the students raise their hands.

Mr. Alexander continues, "How many of you have tried yoga?"

None of the students raise their hands.

"No need to worry. You are going to feel confident practicing yoga by the time you leave today. To start, this is how I can describe yoga to you.

Yoga is a relaxing form of exercise where we hold postures that combine stretching out our limbs and muscles, doing breathing exercises, and using meditation techniques to calm our minds.

Many of us have experienced a "fight-or-flight" feeling. Yoga can help reduce this emotion.

Dr. Garcia introduced the nervous system to your class. Practicing yoga helps move our nervous system from a "fight-or-flight" to "rest-and-digest" feeling.

Additionally, performing yoga exercises helps boost confidence and mindfulness, while also reducing stress."

I am going to teach you one yoga pose before we have to clap our way home.

We are going to learn the "Eagle Pose." Luke and Matthew, please come up to the front with me and copy my movements.

We are going to model this pose for all of you. Please follow our movements:

Stand tall in a mountain pose and wrap one leg around the other.

Next, bring your bent arms out in front of you and wrap your arms together in the opposite way your legs are. Slightly bend your knees.

Mr. Lanci walks around the mats in the park, and says, "They look like professionals already!"

Mr. Alexander proudly speaks up and ends his session with, "Class, I cannot thank you enough for a fun day. Please make sure to keep the *Magic Track* a secret so next year's students can enjoy *Mental Health week*, too! Let's walk one lap around the park on its sidewalk together and enjoy the sounds of nature.

As the class walks together, Cameron is admiring all of the beautiful birds while Olivia is in awe over the variety of plants. The class finished their walk at *Magic Location #4.*

1 clap.
2 claps.
3 claps.

POOF.

<u>Learning Checkpoint #15</u>: <u>In your own words, describe yoga or meditation.</u>

<u>Learning Checkpoint #16</u>: <u>In your own words, describe two mental health benefits from yoga or meditation.</u>

Friday morning

The final day of *Mental Health Week* is here. Once again, the entire class arrived at school before Mr. Lanci. It is a bittersweet moment to say the least.

For Mr. Lanci, he is glad his students are now equipped with information that will help them succeed both inside and outside of the classroom. As Ms. Bridge taught us on Tuesday, he is grateful that the experts were able to take time away from their normal schedules to return to Tampa and interact with his students.

He is sad, however, because this is the last time he will be with this class. He has seen them grow into incredible young men and women with high hopes for all they will accomplish.

To his surprise, Mr. Infeld is leading the students in a morning workout in the field between the teachers parking lot and school entrance. Mr. Lanci walks passed Austin and jokingly says, "You look like you are out of breath!" Austin retorts with, "I am just getting warmed up!"

Mr. Infeld, a University of Tampa (UT) alumnus, decided to stay in Tampa and surprise Mr. Lanci for the final day of the *Mental Health Week*. Since he last joined the class, he has been spending time visiting his favorite restaurants from college and checking out the improvements to UT's campus.

The two teacher's high-five one another and walk the students inside for one more day of fun.

"Staying hydrated is important. Dr. Boccio taught us how our brains need water to function," Luke proudly shares with the class while walking inside.

"We should stop at the water fountain outside the classroom once we walk in. I will hold the door open for everyone."

Stump interferes, "Allow me, Luke," and holds the door open for the class.

Anthony, gasping for breath as he walks up to the fountain, faintly says, "I could do 100 more sit-ups!"

As the class arrives at the cafeteria one last time, Stump takes a class picture. The picture is in the cafeteria, *not* at the *Magic Track*, of course!

For picture day, Mr. Lanci asked his students to wear a shirt that represents their favorite sports team.

Each year, Mr. Lanci's classes become a family after bonding during the final week. The picture taken each *Mental Health Week* is one of a thousand words. Each summer, Mr. Lanci surprises his students by mailing them the picture.

Mr. Lanci wore his green Curtis Martin Jets jersey. Martin was his favorite player growing up. Similar to Mr. Lanci, there were some students wearing football jerseys, too. Paul and Anthony are also wearing Jets jerseys, Charlotte and Mr. Infeld are wearing Giants jerseys, Moses is wearing a Titans jersey, and Jill is wearing a Patriots jersey. The students decided to make silly faces in the picture.

The students have learned so much and still have one more fun-filled day ahead. The class will learn about the importance of giving our minds and bodies a rest when needed. This includes getting enough sleep, taking mental health breaks throughout each day, and prioritizing one day per week as your mental health day ... a day just for you!

"Both the shirt I wore today and *Magic Location #5* have something to do with my Mental Health Day each week. You will find out what that is soon enough," Mr. Lanci says to start the lesson.

"After suffering a Traumatic Brain Injury, certain things became essential for me to succeed. It all starts with getting enough rest each day.

Sleep is very important for children because your brain is still developing. How much sleep are you getting each night?"

"I always sleep at least 10 hours," says Christina.

Gab goes next, "nine hours."

"That is a perfect amount of sleep. Great job, kids. Raise your hand if you like to do well in school?" asks Mr. Lanci.

The whole class raises their hands.

Mr. Lanci's next question is, "Raise your hand if you like to be happy as often as possible."

The whole class puts their hands up.

"You can do well in school and be as happy as possible when you get a good night of sleep. Many of us enjoy watching television shows or movies at night with family, friends, or alone, but it is important to hold ourselves accountable and make sleep a priority.

By getting enough sleep, our attitudes, performance, and quality of life all improve. Now, let's get to why taking a mental health day each week is important.

Taking a mental health day each week if very important not only for adults, but kids, too. We need to rest our brains and bodies from our normal routines to stay mentally and physically healthy.

For you kids, that means no school or homework. You need to take time to do other hobbies and things that make you happy. Shane, what is something that makes you happy that you can do on your mental health day?"

"I love to watch and learn to play golf," says Shane.

"Sports are something that makes me happy, too," follows Mr. Infeld.

Mr. Lanci returns, "On my mental health day, I usually watch or go to a sports game. My favorite teams are the Yankees, Jets, Knicks, and Rangers."

Riley interrupts, "...but Mr. Lanci. What does your football jersey have to with mental health? We still don't know."

"Great timing, Riley. I was about to share. During football season, I use Sunday as my mental health day because that is when the Jets play. Me and my friends growing up have been going to Opening Day, or the first game of the year, since I was a kid. Alex, Alec, Rob, Sam, and I always make great memories at this game.

Lily Rose, what day will be your mental health day next week?"

"I will take my mental health day on Saturday's so I can play soccer in the morning and watch it on the TV in the afternoon," she ecstatically says.

"Now you know what my Jets jersey has to do with my mental health day, but it is time to learn what is has to do with magic.

Everyone, please follow me to the track. We are going to the Jets stadium to get one last group exercise in before we go home for summer. Connor and Paul, please carry the box labeled "Friday" to the *Magic Circle #5*. We will be taking it with us.

You all ready?" The class joyfully screams, "YES", in unison!
1 clap.
2 claps.
3 claps.

POOF.

Learning Checkpoint #17: How many hours of sleep are you going to aim to have each night?

Learning Checkpoint #18: What is a Traumatic Brain Injury?

Friday Afternoon

With only one hour left in the school year, the class arrives at *Magic Location #5*. To be precise, they appear at the 50-yard line on the Jets football field.

"This is where my favorite football team plays. You are going to jog around the field together one time before we head back to the *Magic Track*. You are just like the *pros*.

After you finish jogging, we will enjoy a special lunch. You will be able to eat food from any food vendor you want in the *entire* stadium! Stadium security is spread out around the first floor and they can guide you in any direction. Go!"

As the class jogs together, Mr. Lanci loudly speaks to the class. "We have to do a little learning because this is *still* a school week. Let's have some fun and do some math while you jog.

He yells, "Dana, 9 x 9?"

"81!"

"Jada Joy, 10 x 10?"

"100."

"Lily Mae, please try 11 x 11"

"Hmmm, I think 121?"

Mark, what is 12 x 12?"

"143!

No, excuse me. 144!"

Mr. Lanci claps while sipping his water. He says, "Well done, Mark. Bring it in everyone. Meet at the water table and we will break for lunch. We are going to eat in Section 101."

While the students search the stadium to choose their favorite foods for lunch, Mr. Lanci stands in awe of being on the field. He has been to and watched countless games but has never been on the same field as Curtis Martin.

Spot Check #5: Which will you try first and why? Yoga or meditation?

The students all bring back different foods to their section. Grayson and Bryson both chose chicken tenders with fries. Samantha and Pete chose a cheeseburger and hotdog, respectively.

Mr. Lanci begins to say, "While you are all eating, I am going to teach you about something that helps me succeed each day. Just like taking a day off from our normal schedules, we also need to take breaks during the day. We take breaks so we can rest and take our mind off of what we are working on.

Just as we take a break for a few minutes every hour in the classroom, you need to break outside of school, too.

When we take a break for a few minutes, we can focus better and feel more relaxed. Breaks restore energy in us and help us get through the day easier. Taking breaks helps people with anxiety very much.

"Oh, no!" Mr. Lanci frantically says. "It is 10 minutes past schools ending. Your parents are going to have a lot of questions for you. Remember to always protect our biggest secret."

As the class prepares to leave their final *Magic Location*, Mr. Lanci unwraps Friday's box. "Class, I made these T-shirts for you with our picture from our class trip to New York earlier this year on it. You have made an impact on me and please make sure to visit next year."

1 clap.
2 claps.
3 claps.

POOF.

The class is finally back in Tampa.

The unlikely hero of the week? Stump! When the parents began wondering where their kids were, he covered for them and said, "They are still taking their final exams."

The class hugs Mr. Lanci goodbye, one by one. Tears of happiness are running down the faces of each student. They truly became a *Tampa Family* during *Mental Health Week*.

As the students drive away from *Never Give Up School* for the final time in their lives, Mr. Lanci winks and sends them off to middle school.

"Have a magical summer, kids!"

Learning Checkpoint #19: Describe what you are going to do on your next Mental Health day. Describe this day in at least three complete sentences.

Learning Checkpoint #20: Describe why it is important to take a mental health day in your own words.

Bonus Section

10 activities you can do with family and friends!

1) Colored Candy Go Around

This activity will help you get things off of your chest and can be played with any amount of people. To engage in this activity, you will need to purchase your favorite candy that comes in different colors. Each player starts with seven pieces of candy and the rules for the color of candy are as followed:

- Green – Use words to describe yourself
- Orange – Describe what you can improve in your life
- Red – Describe what worries you
- Yellow – Describe your favorite memories
- Purple – Describe a fun activity you have done with another player

2) Art Class

This is the activity for you if you enjoyed Tuesday of *Mental Health Week* with Ms. Bridge. This activity requires thinking creatively and can be done with any amount of people. With either paint, markers, or crayons, create three pictures.

i.   A picture with your favorite person
ii.   A picture of your favorite food
iii.   A picture describing your favorite hobby

3) Create a "Senses Story"

This activity can be played with up to seven people. It will allow you to tap into your senses by using descriptive words and short phrases to answer the following questions. Afterwards, create either a story, poem, or song with your answers.

1. Where is your favorite place to go?
2. What do you see?
3. What sounds or noises do you hear?
4. What scents or odors do you smell?
5. What are you doing at this location?
6. Who is with you?
7. How does this make you feel?

4) Feelings Hot Potato /Stress Ball

This activity can be done with either balls or potatoes. With this game, play music as the "Stress Balls" are passed around with the players. Whoever has the stress ball when the music stops has to share a memory, idea, or thought on the topic. This is a fun game whether you have a big or small crowd.

5) It is time to cook

This activity is similar to *Activity #2* in that you will need to get creative. Using only five ingredients, you must cook a meal. For each ingredient chosen, each player must share a good quality about each of the other players. Creativity and being supportive for others are a mental health win. Enjoy this game with up to five players.

6) Time to Build a Worry Box

Children experiencing mental health challenges may feel they are controlled by anxious thoughts with difficulty stopping them.

A helpful activity for students struggling with Generalized Anxiety Disorder is to build a "worry box." The student can create and decorate the box however they want.

Adults need to explain to the students that this box is the place in which they keep their worries when they don't want to think about them. This activity will provide kids with a sense of control over their anxiety and adults can choose a certain time of day to talk to kids about their fears.

When they no longer feel as though they need to address a certain worry that is in the box, the piece of paper in the box can be ripped up!

7) Musical Chairs for Feelings

This activity is similar to musical chairs but with a twist! Choose your favorite songs and arrange the chairs in a circle. Next, write feelings words on sticky notes or sticky paper and place them on the chairs.

As the music is playing, each player goes around the room and sits on the chair when the music stops. When each player sits, they call out the word on their chair and the other players give an emotion relating to the name.

8) Reminder or Worry Stones

This activity will help those find comfort who have difficulty separating from someone. It requires oven bake clay and each player to choose three colors that make them feel happy or calm.

Next, each player will roll the colors into a ball. Afterwards, gently push a thumb print into the clay to make it uniquely yours. Discuss what this stone symbolizes for them.

Examples include a positive thought, reminder, or positive mantra like, "I can get through anything."

Bake the clay for 30 minutes at 250 degrees. This stone can be kept in each player's pocket for difficult times as a reminder that things will be okay.

9) Create a Calm Down Jar

This activity requires a jar, preferably plastic to avoid an accident with glass. Fill the jar or container with warm water, glitter, and glitter glue. When times get difficult, shake the jar and watch the glitter float to the bottom. Each player will find this activity to be soothing and an excellent stress reliever.

This is the perfect activity to pair with the breathwork tips you learned with Dr. Garcia. Try deep breathing as you watch the glitter sink to the bottom of the jar and float back up to the top.

10) Activity Log

Throughout this book, you learned that many mental health benefits come from exercise. You also learned the benefits creativity offers. Let's combine both of those. This activity is perfect for two players.

Let's get creative with fitness choices and healthy eating.

For one week, challenge yourself to engage in any form of physical activity for at least 30 minutes with some healthy food to follow.

Track your progress. If you enjoy how you feel after one week, turn it into a lifestyle.

Type of exercise	Number of minutes
Sunday	
Monday	
Tuesday	
Wednesday	
Thursday	
Friday	
Sunday	

Recommended Sleep Chart

Recommended Sleep: 22

0-3 Months Old (Newborn)
- 14-17 hours

4-11 Months Old (Infant)
- 12-15 hours

1-2 Years Old (Toddler)
- 11-14 hours

3-5 Years Old (Preschool)
- 10-13 hours

6-13 Years Old (School-Age)
- 9-11 hours

14-17 Years Old (Teenager)
- 8-10 hours

18-25 Years Old (Young Adult)
- 7-9 hours

26-64 Years Old (Adult)
- 7-9 hours

65+ Years Old (Older Adult)
- 7-8 hours

Glossary

Accountable- subject to the obligation to report, explain, or justify something; responsible; answerable. capable of being explained; explicable; explainable.

Generalized Anxiety Disorder (GAD)- An anxiety disorder characterized by consistent feelings of anxiety for a period of at least six months and accompanied by symptoms such as fatigue, restlessness, irritability and sleep disturbance.

Camaraderie- a spirit of trust and goodwill among people closely associated in an activity or endeavor

Codependent- of or relating to a relationship in which one person is physically or psychologically addicted, as to alcohol or gambling, and the other person is psychologically dependent on the first in an unhealthy way.

Cusp- a point that marks the beginning of a change:

Entrepreneur- a person who organizes and manages any enterprise, especially a business, usually with considerable initiative and risk.

Independent- not dependent; not depending or contingent upon something else for existence, operation, etc.

Immense- vast; huge; very great:

Works Cited

1. "Anxiety Disorders", reviewed by D'Arcy Lyness, PhD in "KidsHealth", https://kidshealth.org/en/parents/anxiety-disorders.html#:~:text=They%20might%20act%20scared%20or,jittery%2C%20or%20short%20of%20breath.

2. "Depression", reviewed by D'Arcy Lyness, PhD in "KidsHealth", https://kidshealth.org/en/parents/understanding-depression.html

3. "31 Tips To Boost Your Mental Health" in "Mental Health America", https://www.mhanational.org/31-tips-boost-your-mental-health

4. "Here's How Creativity Actually Improves Your Mental Health", contributed to by Ashley Stahl, in "Forbes", a. https://www.forbes.com/sites/ashleystahl/2018/07/25/heres-how-creativity-actually-improves-your-health/#3746944713a6

5. "The Importance of Being Grateful", by Deborah Jepsen in "Melbourne Child Psychology & School Psychology Services", https://www.melbournechildpsychology.com.au/blog/importance-grateful/

6. "Creativity and Play: Fostering Creativity", in PBS,
https://www.pbs.org/wholechild/providers/play.html
#:~:text=A%20child's%20cre
ative%20activity%20can,of%20thinking%20and%20p
roblem%2Dsolving

7. "The Foods We Eat Do Affect Our Mental Health.
Here's the Proof.", in Psychology Today,
https://www.psychologytoday.com/us/blog/evidence
-based-living/202001/the-foods-we-eat-do-affect-
our-mental-health-heres-the-proof

8. "Water, Depression, and Anxiety", reviewed by
Mary L. Gavin, MD, in "Solara Mental Health",
https://solaramentalhealth.com/can-drinking-
enough-water-help-my-depression-and-anxiety/

9. "Why Exercise is Good for Your Mental Health", by
Christopher Morh, PhD, RD, in EatingWell,
http://www.eatingwell.com/article/7822525/mental-
benefits-of-exercise/

10. "What Is Psychiatry?", American Psychiatric
Association
a. https://www.psychiatry.org/patients-
families/what-is-psychiatry-menu
12. "Meditation Definition: What is Meditation? Take
Care of the Mind", in MindWorks,
https://mindworks.org/blog/meditation-definition/

13. "Medical Definition of Yoga", by William C. Shiel
Jr., MD, FACP, FACR, in MedicineNet,

https://www.medicinenet.com/script/main/art.asp?a
rticlekey=10811

14. "The Benefits of Meditation For Kids", Thrive
Global, https://thriveglobal.com/stories/the-benefits-
of-meditation-for-kids/

15. "5 Ways Yoga Benefits Your Mental Health", by
Jennifer D'Angelo Friedman, in Yoga Journal,
https://www.yogajournal.com/lifestyle/5-ways-yoga-
is-good-for-your-mental-health

16. "Sleep and mental health: Sleep deprivation can
affect your mental health", in Harvard Health
Publishing: Harvard Medical School,
https://www.health.harvard.edu/newsletter_article/s
leep-and-mental-health

17. "The Importance of Taking Breaks", in "The Well
Being Thesis",
https://thewellbeingthesis.org.uk/foundations-for-
success/importance-of-taking- breaks-and-having-
other-
interests/#:~:text=Taking%20breaks%20has%20bee
n%20shown,and%20cardiovascular%20disease%20%
5B2%5D.

18. "Severe Traumatic Brain Injury Factsheet (for
Schools)" reviewed by Mary L. Gavin, MD in
"KidsHealth", https://kidshealth.org/en/parents/tbi-
factsheet.html#:~:text=A%20severe%20traumatic%2

0brain%20injury,temporary%20effect%20on%20brain%20function

19. "Adult ADHD and Exercise", in WebMD, https://www.webmd.com/add-adhd/adult-adhd-and-exercise

20. "Healthy Foods for Kids", Jeanne Segal Ph.D & Lawrence Robinson in "HelpGuide", https://www.helpguide.org/articles/healthy-eating/healthy-food-for-kids.htm

21. How Much Sleep Do We Really Need?, in Sleep Foundation, https://www.sleepfoundation.org/articles/how-much-sleep-do-we-really-need

22. "The Five Senses", in MentalHealth.net: An American Addiction Centers Resource, https://www.mentalhelp.net/depression/the-five-senses/,

23. "Myers Briggs"
a. https://www.myersbriggs.org/my-mbti-personality-type/mbti-basics/

24. "The Mental Health Benefits of Religion and Spirtuality", in NAMI
a. https://www.nami.org/Blogs/NAMI-Blog/December-2016/The-Mental-Health- Benefits-of-Religion-Spiritual

25. "Depression", in Medline Plus, https://medlineplus.gov/dehydration.html

26. "6 Tips for Teaching Yoga To Beginners", in Yoga National, https://yogainternational.com/article/view/6-tips-for-teaching-yoga-to-beginners

27. "Meditation for Beginners", in Headspace, https://www.headspace.com/meditation/meditation-for-beginners

28. Your Anxiety Loves Sugar. Eat These 3 Things Instead", https://www.healthline.com/health/mental-health/how-sugar-harms-mental-health#withdrawal

29. "Alcohol and Mental Health, in MentalHealth.Org, https://www.mentalhealth.org.uk/a-to-z/a/alcohol-and-mental-health

30. "How to Meditate", in Mindful, https://www.mindful.org/how-to-meditate/

31. "Grateful", in Dictionary.com, https://www.dictionary.com/browse/grateful

32. "Psychologist", in Dictionary.com, https://www.merriam-webster.com/dictionary/psychologist

33. "Breathwork for Children", in Therapy Route, https://www.therapyroute.com/article/breathwork-for-children-by-c-richards

24. "ADHD", in Kids Health, https://kidshealth.org/en/parents/adhd.html#:~:text=ADHD%20stands%20for%20attention%20deficit,at%20home%2C%20and%20in%20friendships

35. "Mental Benefits of Walking, in Jump Start by WebMD, https://www.webmd.com/fitness-exercise/mental-benefits-of-walking#1

36. "10 Family Therapy Activities", in Core Wellness, https://www.corewellceu.com/blog/10-family-therapy-activities/

37. "10 Therapy (and Child)-Approved Activities to support kids with anxiety", in Family Therapy Basics, https://familytherapybasics.com/blog/2017/10/8/10-therapist-and-child-approved-activities-to-support-kids-with-anxiety

38. "Accountable", in Dictionary.com, https://www.dictionary.com/browse/accountable

39. "Generalized Anxiety Disorder", in Dictionary.com, https://www.dictionary.com/browse/generalized-anxiety-disorder

40. "Camaraderie", in Dictionary.com,
https://www.dictionary.com/browse/camaraderie

41. "Codependent", in Dictionary.com,
https://www.dictionary.com/browse/codependent

42. "Cusp", in Dictionary.com,
https://www.dictionary.com/browse/cusp

43. "Independent", in Dictionary.com,
https://www.dictionary.com/browse/independent#

44. "Immense", in Dictionary.com,
https://www.dictionary.com/browse/immense

45. "Entrepreneur", in Dictionary.com,

www.ingramcontent.com/pod-product-compliance
Lightning Source LLC
Chambersburg PA
CBHW050655270326
41927CB00012B/3045